Quinoa Recipes for Rapid Weight Loss

42 Delicious, Quick & Easy Recipes to Help Melt Your Damn Stubborn Fat Away!

Disclaimer

This document is geared towards providing exact and reliable information in regards to the topic and issue covered. The publication is sold with the idea that the publisher is not required to render accounting, officially permitted, or otherwise, qualified services. If advice is necessary, legal or professional, a practiced individual in the profession should be ordered.

- From a Declaration of Principles which was accepted and approved equally by a Committee of the American Bar Association and a Committee of Publishers and Associations.

About This Book

This book aims to introduce you to 42 recipe possibilities incorporating the popular and nutritious South American grain quinoa. It's informational and to the point, and organized into sections on breakfast recipes, meat and fish recipes, vegetarian and vegan recipes, salads, and snack and dessert recipes so you won't be missing any meals! Each section is complete with the needed information.

You will find concluding remarks and a list of resources for additional recipes at the end of this book. I will also give you a preview of another book of mine which I am sure will delight you as well.

The following table of contents will show you exactly what is covered in this book.

Table of Contents

Introduction

Quinoa is a natural grain originating in the Andes Mountains of South America, where it's been eaten for over 3,000 years. It's a superfood that's a complete protein source and rich in the B vitamins as well as vitamin E, iron, magnesium, phosphorus, zinc and pantothenic acid. Besides that, it's easy to digest, gluten-free, and has a low glycemic index. Best of all for weight-loss purposes, it has far fewer calories than better-known grains such as wheat! Quinoa is also extremely versatile in the kitchen, as you'll see from the multitude of healthy and delicious recipes that follow.

Breakfast Recipes

Note: The numbers after the recipes refer to our sources for the recipes. See the <u>Helpful Resources</u> section toward the end of the book.

Banana Berry Smoothie (1)

You can drink this smoothie as a breakfast drink or as a snack. This recipe yields two cups.

Servings: 2

Prep Time: 5 minutes

Cooking Time: 20 minutes

Ingredients

- ½ cup cooked quinoa (cook according to package and chill)
- 1 frozen banana (pre-sliced)
- 1 cup frozen raspberries
- 1½ cups green tea (home brewed without added sweeteners is best), add more or less depending on consistency preferred.
- 6 ice cubes

Directions

1. Put all the ingredients into a blender and blend them until smooth.

Nutritional Components per Serving

- Calories: 328
- Total Fat: 3 g
- Saturated Fat: 0 g
- Trans-fat: 0 g
- Cholesterol: 0 mg
- Sodium: 4 mg
- Carbohydrates: 72 g
- Sugars: 34 g
- Protein: 7 g
- Fiber: 10 g

Breakfast Cereal (1)

You can add any of several topping to make this cereal even yummier: dried apricots, raisins, sliced bananas, diced almonds or walnuts.

Servings: 4

Prep Time: 5 minutes

Cooking Time: 15 minutes

Ingredients

- 1 cup dry white quinoa, pre-rinsed
- 2 cups water
- Kosher or sea salt to taste
- 1 tablespoon honey, optional maple syrup, coconut palm sugar or sucanat
- ½ cup low-fat milk (warmed), optional almond or soy milk

Directions

1. Put the quinoa, water, salt and sweetener into a large saucepan, and stir to combine.

2. Bring to a boil, reduce heat to a low-boil and continue cooking until water has been absorbed, which takes about 15 minutes.

3. Serve with milk.

Nutritional components per serving

- Calories: 185
- Total Fat: 3 g
- Saturated Fat: 0 g
- Trans-fat: 0 g
- Cholesterol: 1 mg
- Sodium: 37 mg
- Carbohydrates: 33 g
- Sugars: 6 g
- Protein: 7 g
- Fiber: 3 g

Blueberry and Walnut Quinoa (2)

A tasty, high-protein change of pace from oatmeal. Lots of vitamins, minerals, antioxidants and other nutrients.

Servings: 2

Prep Time: 10 minutes

Cooking Time: 15 minutes

Ingredients

- ½ cup dry quinoa, rinsed
- 1 cup milk (or almond, soy, etc)
- ¼ cup fresh blueberries
- 1 tablespoon chopped walnuts
- 1 teaspoon cinnamon

Directions

1. Rinse quinoa in a fine mesh strainer, then drain.

2. Combine quinoa and milk in a medium saucepan, and bring to boiling on high heat. Cover and reduce heat to a simmer.

3. Cook 10 to 15 minutes, until the water is absorbed and the quinoa is tender.

4. Stir in the walnuts and cinnamon, and let cool.

5. Add the blueberries on top.

Nutritional components per serving

- Calories: 184
- Total Fat: 5 g
- Sodium: 2 mg
- Carbohydrates: 30 g
- Protein: 7 g
- Fiber: 4 g

Pancakes (3)

If you can't find a place to buy quinoa flour, you can grind or process your own. This is a quick and easy recipe, and you can choose from a multitude of toppings for these pancakes.

Servings: 4 (12 pancakes)

Prep Time: 10

Cooking Time: 20

Ingredients

- 2 cups organic quinoa flour
- 4 teaspoons baking powder
- ½ teaspoon sea salt
- 2 cups plus 1 tablespoon water
- 2 tablespoons vegetable oil

Directions

1. Preheat griddle.

2. Mix the dry ingredients in a bowl.

3. Add the liquid ingredients.

4. Spoon the batter onto the preheated grill, sizing them at 4-5 inches in diameter.

5. Turn the pancakes when the edges seem dry (since they don't contain sugar, the pancakes won't brown very much).

6. If the batter thickens too much while it stands, thin it with 1-2 tablespoons of water.

Nutritional components per serving

- Calories: 182
- Total Fat: 9 g
- Cholesterol: 0 mg
- Sodium: 789 mg
- Carbohydrates: 22 g
- Protein: 4 g
- Fiber: 4 g

Quinoa-crusted Quiche (6)

You can make this ultra-yummy breakfast a mainstay or save it for special occasions.

Servings: 8

Prep Time: 10

Cooking Time: 45

Ingredients

- 1½ tablespoons extra virgin olive oil
- 1 small onion, diced
- 1 small carrot, diced
- 1 red bell pepper, diced
- ¼ cup cooked quinoa
- 2 cups broccoli florets
- 10 eggs, beaten
- 1½ cups unsweetened soy milk
- 2 tablespoons fresh thyme leaves
- ½ teaspoon salt
- 1 pinch black pepper

Directions

1. Preheat oven to 350 F. Lightly oil a 9 x 13-inch baking dish.

2. Heat the olive oil over medium heat in a medium-sized sauté pan. Add the onions carrots and peppers, and sauté until the veggies are tender and the onions are starting to brown. Remove from heat and allow to cool for a few minutes.

3. In a large bowl, combine all the ingredients. Put them into the prepared baking dish and bake for 40 minutes or until the eggs are set.

4. Allow to cool for 5 minutes and serve.

Nutritional components per serving

- Calories: 195
- Total Fat: 10 g
- Cholesterol: 233 mg
- Sodium: 254 mg
- Carbohydrates: 16 g
- Protein: 12 g
- Fiber: 3 g

Quinoa Granola (10)

This granola makes a handy snack or a quick and filling breakfast. You can experiment with substitute nuts and dried fruit. If you want to cut back some on the calories, reduce the amount of coconut oil.

Servings: 6

Prep Time: 10

Cooking Time: 45

Ingredients

- 1 cup rolled oats
- ½ cup quinoa
- ½ cup raw almonds
- ½ cup raw walnuts
- ¼ cup shredded coconut flakes
- ½ cup raisins
- ½ teaspoon cinnamon
- ¼ teaspoon salt
- ¼ cup pure maple syrup
- ¼ cup coconut oil or butter, melted

Directions

1. Preheat oven to 300 degrees. Line a baking pan with parchment paper.

2. Combine all the ingredients in a large bowl or plastic bag, mixing well.

3. Bake for about 45 minutes, until fragrant and lightly browned. Once it's cool, store in an airtight container.

Nutritional components per serving

- Calories: 367
- Total Fat: 22 g
- Sodium: 61 mg
- Carbohydrates: 41 g
- Sugars: 16 g
- Protein: 7 g

Meat and Fish Recipes

Shrimp Paella (1)

This recipe is an adaptation of classic Spanish Paella, substituting quinoa for the rice. Though you can substitute turmeric for the saffron, saffron has a distinctly Spanish flavor that is perfect for this dish.

Servings: 7

Prep Time: 15 minutes

Cooking Time: 30 minutes

Ingredients

- 1 yellow onion, diced
- 2 cloves garlic, minced
- 1 tablespoon olive oil
- 1 ½ cups dry quinoa, rinsed well
- 2½ cups water
- 3 cups chicken broth, fat-free, low-sodium
- ¼ teaspoon crushed red pepper flakes
- 1 bay leaf
- ½ teaspoon saffron threads (or turmeric)
- ½ teaspoon Spanish paprika
- ½ teaspoon black pepper
- Kosher or sea salt to taste
- ½ cup sliced sun-dried tomatoes, packed in olive oil
- 1 red bell pepper, cored, seeded & membrane removed, sliced into 1/2" strips
- 1 cup frozen green peas
- 1 teaspoon seafood seasoning

- 1 pound large shrimp, peeled and deveined, thawed

Directions

1. Put quinoa and water in a medium-sized pot. Cover, bring to a boil and reduce heat to a low-boil. Cook until the quinoa has absorbed most of the water, about 12-15 minutes. Turn the heat off and leave the quinoa on the burner for 5 minutes.

2. Meanwhile, sprinkle shrimp with a pinch of salt and refrigerate it.

3. While quinoa is cooking, heat oil in a large skillet on medium-low. Sauté the onions until tender, about 5 minutes. Add sliced bell pepper strips and sauté an additional 4 minutes. Add garlic and sauté 1 minute.

4. Add the quinoa, chicken broth, red pepper flakes, bay leaves, saffron, paprika, black pepper and salt. Cover and bring to a boil. Reduce heat to a low boil, and continuing cooking for about 10 minutes or until most of the liquid has been absorbed.

5. Add the sun-dried tomatoes, peas and shrimp. Cover and continue cooking for 5 minutes. Remove from heat, leave covered and allow to sit for 10 minutes.

6. Remove the bay leaf and serve.

Nutritional components per serving (1 cup)

- Calories: 273
- Total Fat: 6 g
- Saturated Fat: 1 g
- Trans-fat: 0 g

- Cholesterol: 125 mg
- Sodium: 412 mg
- Carbohydrates: 33 g
- Sugars: 3 g
- Protein: 22 g
- Fiber: 5 g

Skillet Chicken (1)

For this delicious feast, you only need a single pan, so clean-up is a breeze.

Servings: 6

Prep Time: 10 minutes

Cooking Time: 25 minutes

Ingredients

- 6 chicken drumsticks, skin removed (optional breast fillets)
- 1 tablespoon olive oil
- 1 small yellow onion, diced
- 1 clove garlic, minced
- 1 can (14.5 ounces) diced tomatoes in juice
- 2 teaspoons capers, drained
- 1 teaspoon dried oregano
- ½ teaspoon crushed red pepper flakes
- Kosher or sea salt to taste
- ½ teaspoon freshly ground pepper
- ¾ cup chicken broth, fat free, low sodium
- 2 cups cooked quinoa

Directions

1. Put oil in a large non-stick skillet on medium-high heat. Add chicken, browning it on both sides, about 5 minutes per side. Remove chicken and place on a plate lined with a paper towel.

2. Put onion in the skillet, reduce heat to medium-low. Sauté until tender, about 4 minutes. Add garlic and sauté 1 minute.

3. Return chicken to skillet and add the remaining ingredients. Cover and cook until chicken is cooked through and quinoa is tender and has absorbed most of the liquid, about 15 minutes.

Nutritional components per serving

- Calories: 294
- Total Fat: 10 g
- Saturated Fat: 2 g
- Trans-fat: 0 g
- Cholesterol: 90 mg
- Sodium: 145 mg
- Carbohydrates: 19 g
- Sugars: 2 g
- Protein: 30 g
- Fiber: 3 g

Low-carb Cabbage Rolls (2)

These delicious rolls are packed with glutamine (which is important for digestion and muscle health), vitamin C and vitamin A.

Servings: 6 (12 rolls)

Prep Time: 20 minutes

Cooking Time: 50 minutes

Ingredients

- *For the rolls:*
- 12 cabbage leaves
- 1 pound ground chicken
- ¾ cup cooked quinoa
- 1 cup finely chopped red onion
- 1 egg
- ½ cup skim or 1% milk
- 1 teaspoon black pepper
- 2 tablespoons cornstarch
- *For the sauce:*
- 2 cups diced tomatoes
- 1 cup low-sodium tomato sauce
- 1 tablespoon basil
- 2 tablespoons vinegar
- ½ cup chicken broth

Directions

1. Preheat oven to 400 F.

2. Boil or steam cabbage for three minutes in a large pot.

19

3. Combine the chicken, quinoa, onion, egg, milk and pepper in a large bowl, mixing them well.

4. Divide the mixture into twelve equal portions and put each portion on a cabbage leaf.

5. Roll up each cabbage leaf and secure each with a toothpick. Put cabbage rolls side-by-side in a two-inch deep (or deeper) baking dish.

6. Put all the ingredients for the sauce into a bowl, mixing them well. Pour the sauce over the cabbage rolls.

7. Cover the baking dish and set it into the oven, baking for 40 minutes.

8. Remove the cabbage rolls from the baking dish. Transfer the juices from the dish into a saucepan.

9. Mix the cornstarch with ¼ cup cold water in a bowl. Stir this into the juices. Bring to boil, then reduce heat and simmer until the sauce thickens. Pour this sauce over the cabbage rolls when serving them.

Nutritional components per serving (2 rolls)

- Calories: 247
- Total Fat: 11 g
- Saturated Fat: 3 g
- Trans-fat: 0 g
- Sodium: 146 mg
- Carbohydrates: 22 g
- Protein: 22 g
- Fiber: 5 g

Meatloaf Muffins (3)

What kid wouldn't love a giant meatball? These muffins are handy, versatile and unique. You can use two pounds of turkey instead of one pound of turkey and one of beef.

Servings: 12

Prep Time: 30

Cooking Time: 20

Ingredients

- 1 pound ground turkey
- 1 pound lean ground beef
- ½ cup raisins, chopped
- 2 cups of cooked quinoa
- 1 cup of grated or minced carrots
- 1 small onion, minced
- 1/3 cup of an egg substitute (e.g. EggBeaters)
- Dash of milk
- 2 teaspoons Worcestershire Sauce
- Large pinch of oregano
- Salt
- Pepper

Directions

Preheat oven to 450 F.

1. Combine the meats, raisins, quinoa, carrots, onions, salt, pepper, oregano and Worcestershire sauce together, mixing them well. Add the egg substitute and milk, making sure everything holds together.

21

2. Distribute the meat mixture evenly into each cup of an ungreased muffin tin, mounding it a little on top.

3. Bake in your oven for 20 minutes or until done, making sure to cook them completely.

Nutritional components per serving

- Calories: 281
- Total Fat: 11 g
- Cholesterol: 53 mg
- Sodium: 104 mg
- Carbohydrates: 25 g
- Protein: 20 g
- Fiber: 3 g

Chicken and Tomatoes (3)

A filling meal that goes great with a salad.

Servings: 6

Prep Time: 10

Cooking Time: 40

Ingredients

- ½ cup of uncooked quinoa
- 1 can of organic diced tomatoes (no salt added)
- 1 can of chicken broth
- ½ cup of water
- 4 chicken breasts (no skin or bone)
- 2 cloves of garlic (chopped)
- 1 teaspoon salt
- 1 tablespoon black pepper

Directions

1. Put uncooked quinoa in a large saucepan treated with cooking spray (or use a small amount of olive oil). Stir continually until the quinoa has toasted. When quinoa has browned, add chicken stock and water to the quinoa mixture. Allow the mixture to boil, then turn the heat to medium. Cover and cook 10-15 minutes until quinoa is fluffy.

2. While quinoa is cooking, cook the chicken breasts in a skillet until there is no longer pink in the middle.

3. When quinoa and chicken are done, put the chicken in the same pot with the quinoa and add the can of diced

tomatoes, cloves of garlic, salt and pepper. Reduce heat to low and continue mixing ingredients until well mixed. Leave mixed ingredients on low heat for 3-5 minutes to combine the flavors and reduce the excess liquid from the tomatoes. Serve immediately after cooked.

Nutritional components per serving

- Calories: 302
- Total Fat: 4 g
- Cholesterol: 92 mg
- Sodium: 827 mg
- Carbohydrates: 22 g
- Protein: 43 g
- Fiber: 3 g

Pasta-less Pasta Salad (3)

If someone in your family is giving up pasta, they won't miss their pasta after trying this dish. You can add a number of ingredients to this versatile dish, such as broccoli, cauliflower, onion, bell pepper or cucumber.

Servings: 10

Prep Time: 25

Cooking Time: 10

Ingredients

- 1 cup dry quinoa, rinsed
- 2 cups water
- 1 cup cherry tomatoes, halved
- ¼ cup green olives, sliced in half
- 4 ounces cheddar or mozzarella cheese, cut into small cubes
- 1½ ounces pepperoni, quartered
- 1/3 cup Light Italian Dressing

Directions

1. Put quinoa and water in a medium-sized pot. Cover, bring to a boil and reduce heat to a low-boil. Cook until the quinoa has absorbed most of the water, about 12-15 minutes. Turn the heat off and leave the quinoa on the burner for 5 minutes.

2. Put the quinoa into a serving dish. Add the remaining ingredients and toss.

3. Refrigerate for 3-4 hours before serving.

Nutritional components per serving

- Calories: 210
- Total Fat: 10 g
- Cholesterol: 17 mg
- Sodium: 299 mg
- Carbohydrates: 23 g
- Protein: 8 g
- Fiber: 3 g

Vegetarian and Vegan Recipes

Lentil Burgers (1)

Making your own bean burgers is fun and easy, and you can experiment by using a wide variety of toppings for them, such as sautéed mushrooms, tomato, onions, lettuce, ketchup, hummus, guacamole, brie, sprouts, cheese, blue cheese, etc.

Servings: 4 (4 patties)

Prep Time: 10 minutes

Cooking Time: 15 minutes

Ingredients

- 2 tablespoons Dijon mustard
- 3 teaspoons honey
- 1 tablespoon plus 2 teaspoons olive oil
- ¼ cup diced red onion
- 1 cup cooked quinoa
- 1 cup cooked lentils, drained
- 1 can (4-ounce) diced green chilies
- 1/3 cup rolled oats
- ¼ cup whole wheat flour
- 2 teaspoons cornstarch
- ¼ cup whole wheat panko bread crumbs
- ¼ teaspoon garlic powder
- ½ teaspoon cumin
- 1 teaspoon paprika
- Salt and pepper to taste

27

Directions

1. Combine the Dijon mustard and honey in a small bowl and refrigerate until ready to use.

2. Sauté onion in 2 teaspoons olive oil until tender, about 4 minutes.

3. Combine the rest of the ingredients except the rest of the olive oil, mixing them well. Form the mixture into 4 burger patties.

4. Put the rest of the olive oil in a large skillet on medium heat. Cook the patties for about 5-6 minutes on each side, until brown.

5. Put the patties on buns and spread the Dijon mustard mixture on them. Serve.

Nutritional components per serving

- Calories: 430
- Total Fat: 9 g
- Saturated Fat: 1 g
- Trans-fat: 0 g
- Cholesterol: 73 mg
- Sodium: 34 mg
- Carbohydrates: 73 g
- Sugars: 4 g
- Protein: 17 g
- Fiber: 13 g

Stuffed Portobello Mushrooms (1)

This delicious dish is perfect for a quick supper at the end of a hectic day.

Servings: 4 (4 mushrooms)

Prep Time: 20 minutes

Cooking Time: 25 minutes

Ingredients

- 1/3 cup dry quinoa, pre-rinsed
- 2/3 cup water
- 4 large Portobello mushrooms, caps removed
- 1 tablespoon olive oil
- 2 tablespoons balsamic vinegar
- ½ teaspoon black pepper
- ¼ teaspoon crushed red pepper flakes
- Kosher or sea salt to taste
- 1 cup diced vine-ripe tomatoes
- ½ cup whole grain bread crumbs
- ¼ cup freshly chopped basil
- ½ cup feta cheese, fat-free

Directions

1. Preheat oven to 375 F.

2. Put quinoa and water in a medium-sized pot. Cover, bring to a boil and reduce heat to a low-boil. Cook until the quinoa has absorbed most of the water, about 12-15 minutes. Turn the heat off and leave the quinoa on the burner for 5 minutes.

3. Meanwhile, place mushrooms gill (open side) up on a cookie sheet. Brush mushrooms with olive oil and evenly drizzle them with balsamic vinegar. Season with salt to taste.

4. Cook mushrooms 10 minutes. Drain excess liquid from mushrooms.

5. Meanwhile, combine the cooked quinoa, black pepper, red pepper flakes, salt, tomatoes, bread crumbs, basil and feta cheese in a medium-sized mixing bowl.

6. Take mushrooms out of the oven and evenly divide quinoa mixture, approximately ½ cup, into each mushroom. Bake 12 minutes or until mushrooms are tender and cheese is melted.

7. Serve immediately or allow to cool slightly.

Nutritional components per serving (1 stuffed mushroom)

- Calories: 251
- Total Fat: 5 g
- Saturated Fat: 1 g
- Trans-fat: 0 g
- Cholesterol: 5 mg
- Sodium: 427 mg
- Carbohydrates: 41 g
- Sugars: 4 g
- Protein: 12 g
- Fiber: 6 g

Tomato Bowl (2)

This makes a relatively quick and complete lunch for two, or can serve as a side dish for four.

Servings: 4 (4 tomato bowls)

Prep Time: 15 minutes

Cooking Time: 30-35 minutes

Ingredients

- ¼ cup quinoa, dry
- ½ cup water, lightly salted
- 1 tablespoon grapeseed oil
- 2 tablespoons pignoli nuts (pine nuts)
- 2 cloves garlic, minced
- 1 cup fresh spinach leaves
- ½ juice of fresh lemon
- ¼ cup grated cheese of your choice
- 4 organic beefsteak tomatoes, top 1 inch sliced off, pulp and seeds scooped out

Directions

1. Boil the quinoa in the salted water until tender, 15-20 minutes. Drain and rinse the quinoa until cold.

2. Heat the oil in a skillet over medium heat. Stir in the pignoli nuts and cook about 2 minutes, until lightly toasted.

3. Stir the garlic in and cook about 2 minutes, until the garlic softens.

4. Stir in the quinoa and spinach, and cook until the quinoa is hot and the spinach has wilted.

5. Stir in the lemon juice and cheese.

6. Meanwhile, put the tomatoes in a baking dish and put their sliced tops back on top of them. Broil them for 5 minutes until they soften slightly, but still remain intact.

7. Take tomatoes out and fill them with the quinoa mix, using the tomatoes as bowls. Serve.

Nutritional components per serving (1 tomato bowl)

- Calories: 155
- Total Fat: 9 g
- Saturated Fat: 2 g
- Trans-fat: g
- Sodium: 82 mg
- Carbohydrates: 15 g
- Protein: 5 g
- Fiber: 2 g

Quinoa and Veggie Soup (2)

You can throw just about any leftover veggies into this versatile soup that's perfect for a hot lunch on a cold day or as an appetizer for supper.

Servings: 6

Prep Time: 20 minutes

Cooking Time: 15 minutes

Ingredients

- 2-3 tablespoons olive oil
- 1 red onion, finely chopped
- 1 jalapeno, finely chopped
- 2 scallions, thinly sliced
- 1 ½ cups finely chopped mixed vegetables (carrot, celery, zucchini, etc.)
- 4 to 6 garlic cloves, minced
- 4 cups cooked quinoa
- 2 quarts vegetable or chicken stock
- 1 cup cubed Monterey jack cheese (optional)
- ½ cup heavy cream
- handful of fresh cilantro, roughly chopped
- salt and freshly ground black pepper (to taste)

Directions

1. Put a medium-sized pot over medium heat. Add olive oil, red onion, jalapeno and a bit of salt, cooking for a few minutes until the red onions start to turn translucent.

2. Add the scallions and mixed vegetables and cook for 2-3 minutes. Add garlic, cook for 30 seconds before adding the quinoa and stock.

3. Bring to a boil and then lower to simmer.

4. Add cheese and the heavy cream and simmer for 2 minutes. Add cilantro and season to taste.

Nutritional components per serving

- Calories: 182
- Total Fat: 13 g
- Saturated Fat: 4 g
- Protein: 4 g
- Fiber: 4 g

Black Bean Burgers (2)

This is a very quick and easy lunch, and is sure to be a hit with any vegetarian, as well as many meat-eaters. They're delightful when served on a whole-wheat bun with garlic lemon mayo, fresh raw spinach, sliced tomato, and caramelized onions.

Servings: 5 (5 patties)

Prep Time: 10 minutes

Cooking Time: 20 minutes (or 40 if starting with uncooked quinoa)

Ingredients

- 1 15-ounce can black beans, well-drained
- ¾ cup cooked quinoa
- ¼ cup finely diced bell pepper
- 2 tablespoons very finely chopped onion
- ½ cup whole-wheat breadcrumbs
- 1 large clove minced garlic
- ½ tablespoon cumin
- ½ teaspoon salt
- 1 teaspoon hot sauce
- 1 egg
- 3 tablespoons olive oil

Directions

1. Preheat oven to 400 F.

2. Mash the black beans with a fork, leaving some beans whole and others half-mashed.

3. Stir in the quinoa, pepper, onion, breadcrumbs, garlic and then seasonings. Stir in the egg.

4. Form into 5 patties.

5. Bake for 20 minutes, flipping the burgers after 10 minutes.

6. Serve on a bun with favorite toppings.

Nutritional components per serving

- Calories: 235
- Total Fat: 5 g
- Protein: 10 g
- Fiber: 11 g

Quinoa and Broccoli Pilaf (2)

This filling pilaf can serve as a full vegetarian lunch or as a side dish for supper. Super fast and easy.

Servings: 6

Prep Time: 10 minutes

Cooking Time: 20 minutes

Ingredients

- 1 tablespoon extra-virgin olive oil
- 1 medium onion, finely diced
- 1 medium head of broccoli (approximately 1lb), cut into florets and washed
- 1 cup quinoa, dry
- 2 ¼ cup low sodium vegetable broth
- 1 teaspoon sea salt
- 1 teaspoon black pepper
- 1 teaspoon paprika

Directions

1. Shred the broccoli florets and stems in a food processor (or dice them finely with a knife).

2. Sauté the onion in a medium-sized saucepan for about 4 minutes on medium heat.

3. Add the broccoli and sauté for 3 minutes.

4. Add the dry quinoa, veggie broth, salt, pepper and paprika. Cover and bring to boil, then reduce to medium heat and simmer for about 10 minutes, until the liquid has been totally absorbed.

Nutritional components per serving

- Calories: 150
- Total Fat: 3 g
- Sodium: 74 mg
- Protein: 7 g
- Fiber: 7 g

Moroccan Couscous (3)

This is a scrumptious side dish with a kick.

Servings: 4

Prep Time: 15

Cooking Time: 20

Ingredients

- ¼ cup quinoa
- 2 cups water
- 1 lemon, juice and zest
- 1 ounce pine nuts, toasted
- 1 ounce dried currants
- 2 dried figs (chopped)
- ½ teaspoon fennel seeds
- ½ teaspoon coriander seeds
- ¼ teaspoon cinnamon
- ¼ teaspoon cumin seeds
- ¼ teaspoon ground cardamom
- ½ teaspoon salt
- ½ teaspoon pepper
- 2 tablespoons fresh parsley, minced

Directions

1. Grind fennel, coriander, cinnamon, cumin, cardamom, salt and pepper together.

2. Rinse quinoa and pour into a pre-heated non-stick pan. Toast for 1 minute. Add the spice mixture, currants and figs, stirring to combine.

3. Add the water and lemon juice, cover, and bring to boil. Reduce to simmer and cook uncovered for about 15 minutes, until quinoa is done and most of the water is evaporated.

4. Let sit for 5 minutes, then fluff with fork and add the parsley and pine nuts. Optionally add 2 tablespoons of mint.

5. Serve.

Nutritional components per serving

- Calories: 203
- Total Fat: 7 g
- Cholesterol: 0 mg
- Sodium: 313 mg
- Carbohydrates: 34 g
- Protein: 6 g
- Fiber: 4 g

Quinoa and Veggies (3)

This simple but flavorful recipe is lightning fast.

Servings: 4

Prep Time: 5 minutes

Cooking Time: 12-15 minutes

Ingredients

- 1 cup quinoa, rinsed
- 2 cups water
- 4 medium carrots, chopped
- 1 zucchini, chopped
- 8 spears fresh asparagus, chopped
- 1 tablespoon rice wine vinegar
- 2 tablespoons olive oil
- 1 teaspoon fresh thyme, leaves removed from stem
- black pepper to taste

Directions

1. Put quinoa and water in a medium-sized pot. Cover, bring to a boil and reduce heat to a low-boil. Cook until the quinoa has absorbed most of the water, about 12-15 minutes. Turn the heat off and leave the quinoa on the burner for 5 minutes.

2. Meanwhile, steam the vegetables for 3-4 minutes, either in a microwave or in a small covered pot with about a half inch of water.

3. While the quinoa is cooking, prepare the vinaigrette. Put the vinegar and thyme in a small bowl and whisk in the oil.

4. Once the quinoa is cooked, fluff it with a fork. Place 3/4 cup of quinoa on each plate. Arrange a quarter of the vegetables over the quinoa and top with about 2 teaspoons of the vinaigrette.

Nutritional components per serving

- Calories: 295
- Total Fat: 13 g
- Cholesterol: 0 mg
- Sodium: 43 mg
- Carbohydrates: 38 g
- Protein: 7 g
- Fiber: 5 g

Black Bean Casserole (3)

The eggs and cheese help this dish provide a delicious and filling meal in itself.

Servings: 8

Prep Time: 10

Cooking Time: 30

Ingredients

- 1 cup cooked quinoa
- 3 cups cooked black beans (or two 15-ounce cans, drained and rinsed)
- 2 large sweet potatoes, shredded
- 1 cup shredded low-fat cheddar cheese
- 1 tablespoon ground cumin
- Liberal pinches of salt and pepper
- 2 eggs
- 1 cup salsa
- 2 tablespoons fresh cilantro, chopped, for garnish

Directions

1. Preheat oven to 350° F.

2. Coat a 9" x 9" casserole dish with nonstick cooking spray.

3. In a large bowl, mix together the quinoa, black beans, sweet potato, ½ cup of the cheese, and the cumin, salt, and pepper.

4. In a small bowl, mix together the eggs and the salsa. Pour the salsa mixture over the quinoa-bean mixture, then pour everything into the coated casserole dish.

5. Sprinkle the remaining cheese over the top and bake, uncovered, for 30 minutes. Garnish with the cilantro.

Nutritional components per serving

- Calories: 205
- Total Fat: 3 g
- Cholesterol: 63 mg
- Sodium: 315 mg
- Carbohydrates: 32 g
- Protein: 14 g
- Fiber: 9 g

Quinoa Primavera (3)

This is a nice, light pilaf with lots of veggies and nutrients.

Servings: 4

Prep Time: 10 minutes

Cooking Time: 20 minutes

Ingredients

- 1 cup quinoa
- 2 cups water
- Salt to taste
- 2 tablespoons extra-virgin olive oil
- 3 garlic cloves, minced
- 1 small carrot, cut into ¼-inch dice (½ cup)
- 1 celery stalk, cut into 1/4-inch dice (½ cup)
- ½ red bell pepper, finely diced (½ cup)
- ½ green bell pepper, finely diced (½ cup)
- ½ cup edamame (or substitute with fresh or frozen peas)
- 2 scallions, white part only, thinly sliced
- Fresh ground black pepper
- ¼ cup parsley, chopped

Directions

1. Put quinoa and water in a medium-sized pot. Cover, bring to a boil and reduce heat to a low-boil. Cook until the quinoa has absorbed most of the water, about 12-15 minutes.

2. Meanwhile, heat olive oil and garlic in a big skillet over medium heat. When the garlic is aromatic, add the carrots and sauté for 1 minute. Stir in the celery, peppers, edamame (or peas), and scallions. Sauté just long enough for the veggies to heat through, about 1-2 minutes. Stir in the hot quinoa and season with salt and black pepper. Stir in the parsley.

3. Serve immediately.

Nutritional components per serving

- Calories: 269
- Total Fat: 10 g
- Cholesterol: 0 mg
- Sodium: 348 mg
- Carbohydrates: 37 g
- Protein: 9 g
- Fiber: 5 g

Quinoa with Red Pepper and Beans (3)

You can serve this as two separate dishes or mix everything together.

Servings: 4

Prep Time: 20

Cooking Time: 20

Ingredients

- 1 cup quinoa
- 2 ½ cups vegetable broth
- 1 teaspoon chopped garlic
- 2 tablespoons chopped ginger
- 3/4 teaspoon whole cumin seed
- 2 medium red bell peppers cut in strips
- 1 large onion cut into thin wedges
- 1 can (19-ounce) black beans drained and rinsed
- ¼ cup chopped cilantro

Directions

1. Rinse quinoa. Bring 2 cups of broth to a boil in saucepan. Add quinoa and return to boil, then reduce heat to low and simmer for 20 minutes.

2. Heat oil over medium heat. Add garlic, ginger, and cumin seeds and cook for 2 minutes. Add peppers and onion, and cook until tender. Stir in the beans and remaining broth and cook for 2 minutes.

3. Fluff the quinoa with a fork and stir in the cilantro. Top it with the pepper mixture.

Nutritional components per serving

- Calories: 317
- Total Fat: 5 g
- Cholesterol: 0 mg
- Sodium: 598 mg
- Carbohydrates: 59 g
- Protein: 12 g
- Fiber: 10 g

Quinoa a la Tricotine (3)

This is a tasty blend of a variety of veggies, herbs and spices.

Servings: 5

Prep Time: 15 minutes

Cooking Time: 15 minutes

Ingredients

- 1 cup quinoa, dry
- 2 cups water
- 1 medium red bell pepper, cut into small cubes
- 1 teaspoon garlic powder
- 1 teaspoon onion flakes
- ½ teaspoon ground cumin
- ½ teaspoon red pepper flakes
- 1 teaspoon dried oregano leaves
- 1 teaspoon dried parsley leaves
- ½ cup salsa (wild)
- Juice of ½ lemon
- 1 tablespoon olive oil

Directions

1. Put quinoa and water in a medium-sized pot. Cover, bring to a boil and reduce heat to a low-boil. Cook until the quinoa has absorbed most of the water, about 12-15 minutes. Turn the heat off and leave the quinoa on the burner for 5 minutes.

2. Meanwhile, mix all the other ingredients in a big bowl.

3. When the quinoa has sufficiently cooled, mix it into the other ingredients.

4. Serve, or chill before serving.

Nutritional components per serving

- Calories: 182
- Total Fat: 5 g
- Cholesterol: 0 mg
- Sodium: 114 mg
- Carbohydrates: 30 g
- Protein: 6 g
- Fiber: 4 g

Quinoa Casserole (3)

For this tasty recipe, you can substitute olive oil for the butter if you want to save on cholesterol.

Servings: 12

Prep Time: 15

Cooking Time: 25

Ingredients

- 1½ cups quinoa, dry
- 3 cups water
- 2 cans black beans
- 1 container fresh spinach (can use frozen, if thawed)
- 1 tablespoon butter
- 1 8-ounce package of 50% light cheddar, grated
- Seasonings of your choice

Directions

1. Put quinoa and water in a medium-sized pot. Cover, bring to a boil and reduce heat to a low-boil. Cook until the quinoa has absorbed most of the water, about 12-15 minutes. Turn the heat off and leave the quinoa on the burner for 5 minutes.

2. Preheat oven to 400 F.

3. Use half of the tablespoon of butter to sauté the spinach.

4. Mix the cooked quinoa, spinach, rinsed black beans, and half of the cheese. Add seasoning to taste.

5. Grease the casserole dish with the other half of the tablespoon of butter.

6. Put mixture into large the casserole dish and spread the rest of the cheese on top.

7. Bake for about 20 minutes.

8. Allow to cool for at least 5 minutes before serving.

Nutritional components per serving

- Calories: 234
- Total Fat: 6 g
- Cholesterol: 12.5 mg
- Sodium: 141 mg
- Carbohydrates: 33 g
- Protein: 15 g
- Fiber: 9 g

Quinoa Tabouleh (3)

This tasty dish is a quick version of tabouleh.

Servings: 4

Prep Time: 10

Cooking Time: 20

Ingredients

- 1 cup quinoa, dry
- 2 cups water
- 2 cups tomatoes, chopped or sliced
- 1 cup parsley, chopped
- ¼ cup red onion, chopped
- Juice of half a lemon (and the zest, if desired)
- Salt and pepper to taste

Directions

1. Put quinoa and water in a medium-sized pot. Cover, bring to a boil and reduce heat to a low-boil. Cook until the quinoa has absorbed most of the water, about 12-15 minutes. Turn the heat off and leave the quinoa on the burner for 5 minutes.

2. Meanwhile, mix the chopped onion, parsley and tomatoes in a large bowl and set aside.

3. In a separate bowl, whisk the lemon juice, zest (if desired), olive oil and pepper to mix them. Pour this mix over the onion mixture.

4. Add the cooked quinoa and chill before serving.

5. You can serve with hummus, pita and olives.

Nutritional components per serving (1¼ cup)

- Calories: 188
- Total Fat: 3 g
- Cholesterol: 0 mg
- Sodium: 172 mg
- Carbohydrates: 36 g
- Protein: 7 g
- Fiber: 4 g

Quinoa with Spinach and Feta Cheese (3)

This dish is short on prep time but not short on taste.

Servings: 2

Prep Time: 5 minutes

Cooking Time: 15-20 minutes

Ingredients

- ½ cup uncooked quinoa
- 1 teaspoon extra virgin olive oil
- 2 cloves garlic, sliced very thin
- 1 cup baby spinach
- 1 ounce feta cheese, crumbled

Directions

1. Put quinoa and water in a medium-sized pot. Cover, bring to a boil and reduce heat to a low-boil. Cook until the quinoa has absorbed most of the water, about 12-15 minutes. Turn the heat off and leave the quinoa on the burner for 5 minutes.

2. Meanwhile, in a skillet, sauté the garlic in the olive oil over medium heat until the edges of the garlic turn just a little bit light brown, and then reduce the heat to low.

3. When the quinoa is cooked, add it to the skillet along with the spinach. Stir it and cook until the spinach wilts.

4. Add the feta cheese and stir it to combine.

Nutritional components per serving

- Calories: 233
- Total Fat: 9 g
- Cholesterol: 13 mg
- Sodium: 176 mg
- Carbohydrates: 32 g
- Protein: 8 g
- Fiber: 3 g

Roasted Quinoa with Kale and Almonds (7)

This quick and easy dish features kale, a nutritional powerhouse.

Servings: 4

Prep Time: 5

Cooking Time: 25

Ingredients

- 1 tablespoon sesame oil
- 1 cup uncooked quinoa, rinsed
- 2 cups kale, chopped into small pieces
- 1¾ cups water
- ½ cup roasted almonds, chopped or slivered

Directions

1. In a medium-sized saucepan, heat the sesame oil on low heat. Add the quinoa and bring medium heat. Sauté for 3-4 minutes, until the quinoa starts to get fragrant.

2. Add the kale and stir to combine. Add the water and bring to a boil. Reduce to a low simmer. Cover, and cook for 12 minutes.

3. Remove from heat and let it sit uncovered for 10 minutes.

4. Add the toasted almonds and serve.

Nutritional components per serving

- Calories: 272
- Total Fat: 12 g
- Cholesterol: 0 mg
- Sodium: 17 mg
- Carbohydrates: 33 g
- Protein: 10 g
- Fiber: 5 g

Black Beans with Quinoa and Walnuts (9)

This extra-filling dish has more calories than others in this book, but hey, we all need to splurge a little now and then on healthy stuff to avoid the urge to binge. Save this for a special day or for after a hard work-out.

Servings: 4

Prep Time: 20

Cooking Time: 20

Ingredients

- 1 cup uncooked quinoa
- ½ cup walnuts, coarsely chopped
- 3 tablespoons extra virgin olive oil, divided
- 2 cloves garlic, thinly sliced
- ½ cup chopped red onion
- ½ teaspoon ground cumin
- 2 medium tomatoes, chopped into 1/3-inch pieces
- 1 tablespoon balsamic vinegar
- 2 (15-ounce) cans low-sodium black beans, drained and rinsed
- ½ cup cilantro, chopped
- ½ teaspoon salt

Directions

1. Put quinoa and water in a medium-sized pot. Cover, bring to a boil and reduce heat to a low-boil. Cook until the quinoa has absorbed most of the water, about 12-15 minutes. Turn the heat off and leave the quinoa on the burner for 5 minutes.

2. Meanwhile, toast the walnuts in a large, non-stick skillet over medium heat, stirring often until lightly brown and aromatic, about 5 minutes. Transfer to a plate to cool.

3. Put 1 tablespoon of oil in a hot skillet, adding garlic and onion. Cook one minute, while stirring. Stir in the cumin and cook until garlic is golden and vegetables are softened, about 4 minutes. Add tomatoes and cook 1 minute, until just warmed through. Stir this mixture into the quinoa.

4. Whisk together the remaining 2 tablespoons of olive oil and balsamic; stir in quinoa, beans, walnuts, cilantro and salt.

Nutritional components per serving

- Calories: 460
- Total Fat: 16 g
- Saturated Fat: 2 g
- Sodium: 486 mg
- Carbohydrates: 62 g
- Protein: 20 g
- Fiber: 17 g

Salads

Caprese Salad (1)

This recipe only takes 15-20 minutes to make, as you can be prepping while the quinoa is cooking.

Servings: 6 (6 cups)

Prep Time: 15 minutes

Cooking Time: 15 minutes (during prep time)

Ingredients

- 1 cup dry quinoa, cooked according to package directions
- 1 can garbanzo beans, drained
- 1 chopped tomatoes
- 1 chopped cucumber
- 2 medium diced cloves garlic
- 5 large or 10 small fresh, sliced basil leaves
- 1 teaspoon grated ginger root
- Juice of 1 lemon
- 2 baby carrots, diced
- 1 cup of broccoli sprouts (optional)
- 1 cup chopped low fat mozzarella cheese (can also use feta cheese)
- Salt & pepper to taste
- Extra-virgin olive oil & balsamic vinegar, to taste

Directions

1. Mix all the ingredients into a large bowl.

2. Refrigerate for a half hour before serving.

Nutritional components per serving

- Calories: 259
- Total Fat: 5 g
- Saturated Fat: 2 g
- Trans-fat: 0 g
- Cholesterol: 4 mg
- Sodium: 436 mg
- Carbohydrates: 40 g
- Sugars: 4 g
- Protein: 12 g
- Fiber: 9 g

Asian Quinoa Salad (2)

This flavorful salad makes a light and fast lunch.

Servings: 4

Prep Time: 15

Cooking Time: 15

Ingredients

- ½ cup quinoa
- ½ cup diced red bell pepper
- ½ cup thinly sliced scallions
- ½ cup diced cucumber
- 3 tablespoon fresh lime juice
- 1 tablespoon olive oil
- 1 teaspoon agave nectar
- ¼ teaspoon fine sea salt
- ¼ teaspoon ground black pepper
- 1 teaspoon black sesame seeds
- ¼ cup fresh cilantro leaves, coarsely chopped

Directions

1. Put the quinoa into a cup of water in a medium saucepan and bring to a boil over high heat. Cover, reduce to a simmer, and cook until the liquid is absorbed, which takes about 15 minutes.

2. Spoon the quinoa into a bowl and fluff it with a fork. Add the bell pepper, scallions, and cucumber, tossing to combine them.

3. In a separate small bowl, whisk together the lime juice, olive oil, agave, salt, and black pepper. Add this mixture to the quinoa mixture and toss well.

4. Top the dish with the sesame seeds and cilantro.

Nutritional components per serving (2/3 cup)

- Calories: 238
- Total Fat: 9 g
- Carbohydrates: 35 g
- Protein: 6 g

Cranberry Salad (3)

A delicious salad that is perfect for picnics. It keeps several days in the fridge.

Servings: 8

Prep Time: 15

Cooking Time: 15

Ingredients

- 3 cups water
- 1 ½ cups quinoa
- 1 clove garlic
- 1 tablespoon lemon juice
- 2 tablespoons olive oil
- 2 tablespoons balsamic vinegar
- 1 ½ cups dried cranberries (craisins)
- 1 cup diced celery
- ¼ cup sunflower seeds
- 1 tablespoon rosemary

Directions

1. Boil the water and add the quinoa. Lower the heat and simmer until most of the water is absorbed (takes about 15 minutes). While it's simmering, add the garlic, lemon and salt.

2. Remove the quinoa from the heat and stir in the oil and vinegar.

3. Toss the quinoa mixture with the celery, sunflower seeds, cranberries and rosemary.

Nutritional components per serving (¾ cup)

- Calories: 251
- Total Fat: 8 g
- Cholesterol: 0 mg
- Sodium: 16 mg
- Carbohydrates: 43 g
- Protein: 6 g
- Fiber: 7 g

Quinoa and Black Bean Salad (3)

This substantial salad provides a delicious and filling meal that is high in protein and other nutrients. You can refrigerate this salad for a day before serving, though the salad only takes a total of 15 minutes or so to make.

Servings: 8

Prep Time: 15 minutes (while quinoa is cooking)

Cooking Time: 15 minutes

Ingredients

- 1½ cups quinoa, dry
- 3 cups water
- 1½ cups canned black beans, rinsed and drained
- ½ tablespoon red wine vinegar
- 1½ cups cooked corn (fresh, canned or frozen)
- 1 red bell pepper, seeded and chopped
- 4 scallions, chopped
- 1 teaspoon garlic, minced fine
- ¼ teaspoon cayenne pepper
- ¼ cup fresh coriander leaves, chopped fine
- 1/3 cup fresh lime juice
- ½ teaspoon salt
- 1¼ teaspoon ground cumin
- 1/3 cup olive oil

Directions

1. Put quinoa and water in a medium-sized pot. Cover, bring to a boil and reduce heat to a low-boil. Cook until the quinoa has absorbed most of the water, about 12-15

minutes. Turn the heat off and leave the quinoa on the burner for 5 minutes.

2. Toss the beans with the vinegar, salt and pepper, in a small bowl. Add the beans, corn, bell pepper, scallions, garlic cayenne and coriander to the pot of quinoa, and toss well.

3. Whisk together the lime juice, salt and cumin, adding a stream of oil while whisking. Drizzle over the salad and toss well with salt and pepper. Bring to room temperature before serving.

Nutritional components per serving

- Calories: 370
- Total Fat: 13 g
- Cholesterol: 0 mg
- Sodium: 210 mg
- Carbohydrates: 55 g
- Protein: 11 g
- Fiber: 8 g

Warm Chicken Salad (3)

This is a super-quick dish that can serve as a complete meal.

Servings: 4

Prep Time: 20 minutes

Cooking Time: 10 minutes

Ingredients

- 1 ½ teaspoon minced garlic
- 2 carrots, shredded
- 1 small zucchini, sliced and quartered
- ½ cup red bell pepper
- 12 ounces diced chicken
- ½ cup chopped scallions
- 2 tablespoons olive oil
- 3 tablespoons vinegar
- ¼ teaspoon salt
- 1 cup cooked quinoa
- 4 cups baby spinach

Directions

1. Heat pan coated with no-stick spray to medium heat. Sauté the garlic, zucchini, carrots, pepper and chicken until the chicken is cooked through and the vegetables are softened, about 7 minutes.

2. Combine the scallions, oil, vinegar, salt and pepper in a food processor or blender, and blend until thick. Add this mixture to the chicken mixture and heat it through.

3. Place one cup of spinach on each plate, and top each with a fourth of the quinoa mixture.

Nutritional components per serving

- Calories: 235
- Total Fat: 8 g
- Cholesterol: 49 mg
- Sodium: 112 mg
- Carbohydrates: 17 g
- Protein: 23 g
- Fiber: 3 g

Pomegranate Salad (3)

A festive side dish for any occasion.

Servings: 8

Prep Time: 15 minutes

Cooking Time: 10 minutes

Ingredients

- 1 ½ cups quinoa, rinsed in cold water
- 3 cups water
- 1 ½ teaspoons kosher salt
- ½ cup scallion greens, sliced into thin rounds
- ½ bunch flat-leaf parsley, roughly chopped
- Seeds from 1 pomegranate (about 1 cup)
- ½ cup toasted sliced or slivered almonds (optional)
- 1 tablespoon extra virgin olive oil
- 1 teaspoon red wine vinegar
- 1 teaspoon granulated sugar
- Kosher salt and ground black pepper to taste

Directions

1. Put quinoa and water in a medium-sized pot. Cover, bring to a boil and reduce heat to a low-boil. Cook until the quinoa has absorbed most of the water, about 12-15 minutes. Turn the heat off and leave the quinoa on the burner for 5 minutes.

2. Mix the rest of the ingredients (except the salt and pepper) in a large bowl.

3. Add the quinoa to the mix and season with salt and pepper.

4. To serve, top with the toasted almonds.

Nutritional components per serving

- Calories: 154
- Total Fat: 6 g
- Cholesterol: 0 mg
- Sodium: 440 mg
- Carbohydrates: 21 g
- Protein: 5 g
- Fiber: 3 g

Greek Quinoa Salad (4)

This delicious recipe is from the American Diabetes Association. The low-carb veggies in this dish add plenty of potassium and other nutrients.

Servings: 10

Prep Time: 15 minutes

Cooking Time: No cooking

Ingredients

Ingredients for the salad:

- 1 cup quinoa
- 2 cups low-sodium, reduced-fat chicken broth (or gluten-free broth)
- 1 large cucumber, peeled, seeded and diced
  - 10 ½ -ounce container grape tomatoes, cut in half
- ¼ cup red onion, finely diced
- ¼ c fresh parsley, chopped
- ½ cup reduced-fat feta cheese, crumbled

Ingredients for the dressing:

- ¼ cup red wine vinegar
- 2 tablespoons olive oil
- ½ tablespoon Dijon mustard
- ½ packet Splenda

Directions

1. Cook quinoa according to package directions, using the chicken broth. Let it cool completely.

2. In a large salad bowl, combine the cooled quinoa with the rest of the salad ingredients.

3. In a small bowl, whisk together dressing ingredients. Pour the dressing over salad and mix to coat. Serve cold.

Nutritional components per serving

- Calories: 115
- Total Fat: 5 g
- Saturated Fat: 1 g
- Cholesterol: 5 mg
- Sodium: 135 mg
- Carbohydrates: 14 g
- Protein: 5 g
- Fiber: 2 g

Quinoa Fruit Salad (5)

This is a refreshing salad that's perfect for hot summer afternoons.

Servings: 6

Prep Time: 15 minutes

Cooking Time: 2 hours in the refrigerator

Ingredients

- ¾ cup plain non-fat Greek yogurt
- 2 tablespoons lime juice, divided
- 5 fresh mint leaves, minced
- 2 cups cooked quinoa
- Optional dash of salt and pepper
    - cup blueberries
- 1 cup green grapes, halved
- ½ cup raspberries
- 1 teaspoon agave nectar

Directions

1. In a small bowl, combine the yogurt, mint and 1 tablespoon of the lime juice. Pour this over the cooked quinoa, mixing it well. Season with salt and pepper to taste.

2. In a separate bowl, combine the fruit, agave nectar and the rest of the lime juice.

3. Cover and refrigerate both bowls for 2 hours.

4. Combine the two bowls and serve.

Nutritional components per serving

- Calories: 114
- Total Fat: 1 g
- Sodium: 13 mg
- Carbohydrates: 20 g
- Protein: 6 g
- Fiber: 3 g

Avocado and Black Bean Salad (8)

If you want a salad that will fill you up with healthy fats, this is your recipe. The avocado, black beans and olive oil will satisfy even the healthiest appetite.

Servings: 4

Prep Time: 5 minutes

Cooking Time: 25 minutes

Ingredients

- cup dry quinoa, rinsed
- ¾ cups water
- ½ red bell pepper, diced
- scallions, thinly sliced
- ¼ cup pumpkin seeds, toasted
- tablespoons extra virgin olive oil
- ¾ tablespoon fresh lime juice
- 1 pinch sea salt
- cups baby arugula
- 1 fresh ripe avocado
- 1 can (15-ounce) black beans, drained and rinsed
- tablespoons fresh cilantro

Directions

1. Put quinoa and water in a medium-sized pot. Cover, bring to a boil and reduce heat to a low boil. Cook until the quinoa has absorbed most of the water, about 12-15 minutes. Turn the heat off and leave the quinoa on the burner for 5 minutes.

2. Add the pepper, scallions and pumpkin seeds to the quinoa.

3. In a small bowl, combine the olive oil, lime juice and salt, then toss them in with the quinoa mixture.

4. To serve, put some of the arugula onto a plate and then spoon some of the quinoa salad on top of it. Garnish with the avocado slices, black beans and cilantro.

Nutritional components per serving

- Calories: 361
- Total Fat: 21 g
- Cholesterol: 0 mg
- Sodium: 103 mg
- Carbohydrates: 36 g
- Protein: 10 g
- Fiber: 8 g

Snack and Dessert Recipes

Meatless Meatballs (1)

You can use this versatile dish as a party favorite, appetizer, snack, lunch or side dish, or incorporate into spaghetti or other pasta dish. These are great for eating prior to working out, because they provide complex carbohydrates (for energy) and protein (for building muscles). For vegan meatballs, substitute vegan egg replacer or 1 tablespoon flax meal mixed with 3 tablespoons of water.

Servings: 4 (8 meatballs)

Prep Time: 20 minutes, plus 2 hours chilling time

Cooking Time: 30-35 minutes

Ingredients

- ½ cup dry quinoa, pre-rinsed
    - cup water
- 1 cup cooked green lentils, well-drained
- ¼ cup diced red bell pepper
- ½ cup diced onion
    - cloves garlic, minced
- ½ cup gluten-free bread crumbs
- ¼ cup freshly grated parmesan
- 1 tablespoon freshly chopped flat parsley leaves
- 1 tablespoon freshly chopped oregano
- ½ teaspoon freshly ground black pepper
- Sea salt to taste
- ¼ teaspoon cayenne pepper
- 1 egg white

o   tablespoons olive oil

Directions

1. Put pre-rinsed quinoa and water into a medium-sized pot. Cover it and bring to a boil. Reduce heat to a simmer and continue cooking 15 minutes or until water is completely absorbed.

2. Meanwhile, put 1 tablespoon olive oil in a large non-stick skillet on medium-low heat and sauté diced onions and bell pepper until tender, about 4 minutes. Add the garlic, parsley and oregano and sauté one additional minute.

3. Remove quinoa from heat and allow to sit 10 minutes. Press down on quinoa with a paper towel to remove any remaining water.

4. In a large mixing bowl combine sautéed onion, garlic, parsley and oregano along with remaining ingredients, except oil. Mash the ingredients well, using either a potato masher or a fork. Roll up the mixture into 1½ inch meatballs. Put them into a large bowl, cover and refrigerate until chilled, about 2 hours.

5. Add the remaining 2 tablespoons of oil to a large non-stick skillet, heat to medium-low and add meatballs. Brown the meatballs on both sides, about 16 minutes total. Remove from skillet and drain the meatballs on a paper towel.

6. If you plan to serve these meatballs with marinara, add to the marinara sauce, gently turning them to coat. Simmer until hot and serve over pasta.

Nutritional components per serving (2 meatballs)

- Calories: 145
- Total Fat: 6 g
- Saturated Fat: 1 g
- Trans-fat: 0 g
- Cholesterol: 2 mg
- Sodium: 59 mg
- Carbohydrates: 19 g
- Sugars: 1 g
- Protein: 8 g
- Fiber: 4 g

Almond Joy Bars (1)

These delicious treats are only 94 calories apiece, with no trans-fat, only two grams of saturated fat and 6 grams of total fat per bar. They make great snacks, or you can use them as a dessert.

Servings: 14 mini bars

Prep Time: 15 minutes

Cooking Time: 20 minutes

Ingredients

- 1/3 cup (dry) quinoa
- 2/3 cup water
- 12 whole dates, no sugar added
- 1/2 cup whole almonds with skins
- 1/3 cup grated coconut (unsweetened)
- 2 - 3 teaspoons water
- ¼ cup dark chocolate chips

Directions

1. Put the quinoa and water into a small, covered saucepan and bring to a boil. Reduce heat and simmer for 15 minutes or until all the water has been absorbed. Cool to room temperature. (If you already have one cup of cooked quinoa available to use for this dish, skip this step.)

2. Refrigerate the quinoa for at least two hours.

3. Put dates into a food processor and pulse them until they form a ball.

4. Add almonds to the dates and pulse them until they're finely minced, but don't turn them into mill.

5. Add the coconut and quinoa to the mixture and pulse until the ingredients are well combined.

6. Put all the ingredients into a mixing bowl and mix in one teaspoon of water at a time until the mixture holds together. Shape the mixture into 14 mini bars or balls.

7. Put the chocolate chips into a small saucepan and melt over low heat, or melt them in a double-boiler.

8. Drizzle warm chocolate over each bar or ball. Refrigerate until the chocolate hardens.

9. For storing the bars or balls, you can refrigerate them in a sealed container for several days or freeze them in a freezer safe dish.

Nutritional components per serving (1 bar)

- Calories: 94
- Total Fat: 6 g
- Saturated Fat: 2 g
- Trans-fat: 0 g
- Cholesterol: 0 g
- Sodium: 2 mg
- Carbohydrates: 10 g
- Sugars: 4 g
- Protein: 2 g
- Fiber: 2 g

Vegan Chocolate Protein Bars (2)

If you're tired of shelling out good money for processed protein bars, now you can make your own with this easy recipe. These yummy bars deliver all the energy you need to fuel a work-out or a busy afternoon.

Servings: 12 (12 bars)

Prep Time: 15 minutes

Cooking Time: 35-40 minutes

Ingredients

- ¾ cup dry quinoa (or about 2 cups cooked)
- ½ cup dates, pitted
- 3 tablespoons agave nectar
- 2 tablespoons vegetable oil
- 2 tablespoons ground flaxseed
- ½ teaspoon almond extract
- ¼ teaspoon salt
- ½ cup protein powder
- ½ cup whole-wheat flour
- ¼ cup shredded coconut
- ¼ cup vegan chocolate chips

Directions

1. Preheat oven to 350 F. Lightly coat an 8x8 baking dish with baking spray.

2. Rinse the quinoa in cold water and then soak it for 10 minutes. Bring 1 cup of water to boil, then drain the quinoa and add it to the boiling water. Cover and

reduce heat, letting the quinoa simmer for about 12 minutes.

3. Let the quinoa cool enough to handle it, and then combine it in a food processor with the dates, agave nectar, oil, flaxseed, almond extract and salt. Process until relatively smooth.

4. In a small bowl, stir the protein powder, flour, shredded coconut and chocolate chips together. Fold this dry mixture into the wet mixture with a spatula. This makes for a thick dough, so you'll need to press this dough into the prepared pan with a spatula to spread it evenly.

5. Bake for 22-25 minutes until firm. Let it cool and then slice it into 12 bars.

6. These bars can be stored in an airtight container for up to a week, or frozen for up to three months.

Nutritional components per serving

- Calories: 184
- Total Fat: 5 g
- Saturated Fat: 3 g
- Trans-fat: 0 g
- Sodium: 37 mg
- Potassium: 113 mg
- Carbohydrates: 29 g
- Protein: 7 g
- Fiber: 3 g

Quinoa Pudding (10)

This is a creamy and delicious alternative to rice pudding. You can serve it with fruit or eat it as is. Sweet and nutritious.

Servings: 6

Prep Time: 10 minutes

Cooking Time: 35-40 minutes

Ingredients

- cup quinoa
- ¼ cup granulated sugar
- ¼ teaspoon ground cardamom
- ¼ teaspoon cinnamon
- ¼ teaspoon salt
- cups skim milk
- 2/3 cup water
- 1 tablespoon pure vanilla extract

Directions

1. Put the quinoa, sugar, spices, milk and water in a medium saucepan and bring to a boil, making sure to watch carefully so it doesn't boil over. Reduce heat to medium low and cover. Simmer for 30 minutes.

2. Remove the lid and stir in the vanilla. If you would like it thicker, simmer for up to 10 more minutes.

3. Remove from heat and allow to cool before serving.

Nutritional components per serving

- Calories: 189
- Total Fat: 2 g
- Sodium: 165 mg
- Carbohydrates: 34 g
- Sugars: 15 g
- Protein: 8 g

Dessert Bars (11)

Though these bars make for an easy and yummy dessert, you can save any leftover bars in the fridge for snacks. If storing for longer than a day or two, put them in the freezer.

Servings: 12 bars

Prep Time: 10

Cooking Time: 50-60

Ingredients

- 2 cups quinoa flakes
- ½ teaspoon nutmeg
- 2 tablespoons finely chopped apricots
- 2 tablespoons desiccated coconut
- 2 whisked egg whites
- 2 tablespoons melted butter
- ½ cup maple sugar
- ¼ cup maple syrup
- 2 teaspoons vanilla essence
- 3 teaspoons cinnamon

Directions

1. Preheat oven to 250 F. Grease an 8-inch square baking pan.

2. Mix all the ingredients together, except for the cinnamon.

3. Press the mixture into the prepared baking pan. Sprinkle the cinnamon on top.

4. Bake 40-50 minutes. Take out of the oven to cut into bars. Put the pan back into the oven to bake for 10 more minutes.

5. Take pan out to cool.

Nutritional components per serving

- Calories: 290
- Total Fat: 8 g
- Sodium: 61 mg
- Carbohydrates: 46 g
- Sugars: 21 g
- Protein: 7 g

Conclusion

This book has provided an introduction to recipe ideas that can help you lose weight and improve your health with the superfood quinoa. You've learned how to take advantage of its high protein and vitamin content, gluten-free status, and low calorie count and glycemic index in recipes that you'll find easy to make and irresistible on your plate.

This book offers 42 easy-to-follow quinoa recipes for shedding pounds and inches while contributing to your physical and mental wellbeing. These recipes are structured in a consistent format that provides the number of servings, prep and cooking time for each recipe, as well as the nutritional components per serving. The directions are thorough, clear and concise. The dishes are varied, covered a broad base of foods, giving you a well-balanced selection of foods to choose from.

These 42 delicious quinoa recipes are just a start. Through them, you'll be able to better understand how you can substitute quinoa for many of the other grains in your existing recipes from other sources. This expansion of your food choices can lead you and your family to not only trimmer figures, but also a fuller, healthier and happier life.

Helpful Resources

1. SkinnyMs

2. *The Everything Wheat-Free Diet Cookbook: Simple, Healthy Recipes for Your Wheat-Free Lifestyle* by Lauren Kelly

3. Recipe Bridge

4. American Diabetes Association

5. Narayan Wellness

6. *The Great Cholesterol Myth Cookbook* by Jonny Bowden et al.

7. Dr. Mark Hyman

8. Whole Foods Market

9. Tiny Farmhouse

10. whole living

11. Fitness Foodie

Preview of Gluten Free Diet Guide: A Blueprint to Jump Starting a Healthy, Low Budget, Gluten-Free Diet

Background

Gluten is a protein compound present in cereal grains such as wheat, rye and barley. Gluten is a Latin word which translates to "glue," referring to the combined water-insoluble proteins, gliadin and glutenin. Gluten is the substance that makes dough elastic and processed food items like bread, pasta and pastries chewy. This substance may also be present in cosmetics such as make-up and hair products.

A significant percentage of the population in North America have sensitivity to gluten where they experience an elevated immunologic response when they ingest foods that contain gluten. This usually leads to symptoms such as joint pain, anemia, tiredness, infertility, neurological disorders, dermatitis, and celiac disease, an autoimmune disorder.

The only known treatment for these health issues is to totally embrace a gluten-free diet. This means the person has to steer clear of foods that contain rye, barley, wheat, and other associated cereal grains. Because of the popularity of these grains in the food market, it is possible that items claiming to be gluten-free may have minute amounts of wheat, rye, or barley that is substantial enough to cause symptoms to persons that are sensitive to gluten.

Symptoms and disorders caused by gluten-containing food items

A review from the New England Journal of Medicine came up with a listing of illnesses caused by ingestion of gluten. Symptoms include Attention Deficit Hyperactivity Disorder (ADHD), anxiety, arthritis, depression, Irritable Bowel Syndrome (IBS), recurrent headaches, osteoporosis, eczema, fatigue, uncoordinated muscles, compromised immune system, inflammation of organs, excessive growth of fungus, weight loss or weight gain, and deficient nutrition. People who are hypersensitive to gluten are at high risk to develop diabetes, Gastro-Intestinal cancers, obesity, brain disorders, thyroid problems, and autism.

Costs involved with a gluten-free diet

A recent study assessed the economic burden of subscribing to a total gluten-free diet. The researchers conducted an analysis of food products that use wheat classified by brand name, size or weight of the package, and evaluated them in contrast to items that are gluten-free. The price disparities were also evaluated among different store venues like general stores, more expensive grocery stores, health food stores, and online grocery sites.

The study found that availability of gluten-free products varies among stores. General grocery stores offer 36 percent, while upper class grocery stores have 41 percent, and health food stores carry 94 percent in comparison to a hundred percent availability in online grocery sites. On the whole, all gluten-free products were costlier than wheat-based food items. Gluten-free pasta and bread are double the price of wheat-based pastas and breads.

Apparently, the purchase venue had more impact on the price ranges than geographic location. Researchers conclude that gluten-free items are not as available and are costlier than products that contain gluten. The author emphasizes that there is a need to address availability and cost issues of gluten-free foods that affect the dietary adherence and quality of life of gluten-sensitive consumers.

To fully enjoy this book, visit:

http://www.amazon.com/Gluten-Free-Diet-Guide-Blueprint-ebook/dp/B00I135OZO

Did You Like This Book?

Before you leave, I wanted to say thank you again for buying my book.

I know you could have picked from a number of different books on this topic, but you chose this one so I can't thank you enough for doing that and reading until the end.

I'd like to ask you a small favor.

If you enjoyed this book or feel that it has helped you in anyway, then could you please take a minute and post an honest review about it on Amazon?

Click here to post a review.

Your review will help get my book out there to more people and they'll be grateful, as will I.

More Books You Might Like

Household DIY: Save Time and Money with Do It Yourself Hints and Tips on Furniture, Clothes, Pests, Stains, Residues, Odors and More!

DIY Household Hacks: Save Time and Money with Do It Yourself Tips and Tricks for Cleaning Your House

Essential Oils: Essential Oils & Aromatherapy for Beginners: Proven Secrets to Weight Loss, Skin Care, Hair Care & Stress Relief Using Essential Oil Recipes

Apple Cider Vinegar for Beginners: An Apple Cider Vinegar Handbook with Proven Secrets to Natural Weight Loss, Optimum Health and Beautiful Skin

Body Butter Recipes: Proven Formula Secrets to Making All Natural Body Butters that Will Hydrate and Rejuvenate Your Skin

If the links do not work, for whatever reason, you can simply search for these titles on the Amazon website to find them.

www.ingramcontent.com/pod-product-compliance
Lightning Source LLC
Chambersburg PA
CBHW010246030426
42336CB00022B/3323